$$\boxed{O_2 O_2 O_2}$$

OXYGEN

OXYGEN

OXYGEN

HYDROGEN PEROXIDE
MAGNESIUM PEROXIDE
CHLORINE PEROXIDE

Kurt W. Donsbach D.C., Ph.D.

Published by
THE ROCKLAND CORPORATION
©1993

All rights reserved. No part of this book may be reproduced in any form, nor by any means, without specific written permission from the author.

Printed in USA

wB995-14

From the Author & Publisher:

This book does not intend to diagnose disease nor to provide specific medical advice. Its intention is solely to inform and to educate. The author and publisher intend that readers will use the information presented in this book in cooperation with a health professional.

FORWARD

This book was written because of a substance that has captured the imagination of people around the world. Hydrogen peroxide is a simple chemical compound containing two elements - hydrogen and oxygen. Of these, it is oxygen which acts as the catalyst, producing the many changes we write about. So this book is really about oxygen, not hydrogen peroxide.

Just as Ford built the first automobile, ushering in a whole new era of transportation, so has hydrogen peroxide focused our attention on the possibilities of using other sources of oxygen than the air we breathe. Just as Ford soon had a multitude of competitors, hydrogen peroxide also has its competitors in the oxygen-bearing chemicals, each with something to offer.

We will discuss my reason for not using many of these substances later, but my work and clinical research at our two hospitals has led me to magnesium peroxide because it is most desirable from a palatability standpoint and is easy to work with.

All of my original research was done with hydrogen peroxide; all of the work done by the great Dr. Rosenow at Mayo Clinic and the work done at Baylor University used hydrogen peroxide. It is still the preferred intravenous infusion product and the one I will continue to use for external applications. For oral ingestion, however, I now believe the product of choice to be magnesium peroxide, and it may have even more to offer. The oxygen content is more stable than that in hydrogen peroxide and when it is chemically reduced, it leaves a very beneficial mineral, magnesium, as oxygen is released.

I have discussed this at length with Wally Grotz and Father Wilhelm, the two people most responsible for my introduction to hydrogen peroxide (oxygen) therapy. Both of them agree with me that magnesium peroxide will do what hydrogen peroxide will and may offer an easier-to-handle-vehicle for oxygen.

Thus it is important that as you read this book, which largely concentrates on hydrogen peroxide research, you always be aware of two factors.

    1. What we are really talking about, the substance that helps achieve the remarkable changes in the human body, is oxygen.

    2. Magnesium peroxide is an excellent oxygen donor and the end result of its oral use is the same as hydrogen peroxide used orally.

Comparison

	%Oxygen	Waste Product	Taste	Stability
H_2O_2	94%	Water	Metallic	Fair
MgO_2	57%	Magnesium	Pleasant	Good

WHICH PEROXIDE SHOULD YOU TAKE?

So much effort has been made to malign hydrogen peroxide that it has gotten to the point where serious, but misinformed would-be journalists are beginning to pick up on these deviations from truth and repeat, under their own byline, erroneous statements that could lead the uninformed down the wrong pathway.

I would be the first to say that the individual should have the freedom of choice to use the oxygen-containing product which they desire. When it comes right to it, the whole debate really boils down to whether you should take chlorine dioxide (chlorine peroxide) or hydrogen dioxide (hydrogen peroxide) or magnesium dioxide (magnesium peroxide). At the present time, these three are the practical choices that an individual has. But the water has become so muddied that most who do any reading are confused. I hope this little missle of facts will put things in proper perspective and prevent further confusion. Let's deal with a few of the issues in a factual form.

Question: Why do so many of the products which are sold as "liquid oxygen" fail to tell you what they really contain? One company would have you believe that they take a juice and pump gaseous oxygen into it, making it the best! That's impossible - pure and simple. Another says that it is a deep and private secret formula dreamed up by a chemist. More hogwash! There are no secret formulas when it comes to oxygen-containing liquids. There are just a few and they are well known. I do know that one of these formulae put out by a certain company was nothing more or less than ordinary laundry bleach, commonly called "Clorox." It is, incidentally, one of the oxygen-containing liquids known to all chemists, but not one that I would choose to consume, even though diluted. Most of the products are a dilution of chlorine dioxide, the most honest name for it being dioxychlor which is a rearrangement of the real name. Let's take a look at chlorine dioxide.

Chlorine dioxide is an oxygen-containing compound, highly unstable, which can be altered by oxidation to several other compounds. Because of its chemical bonding, it cannot release anything otherthan nascent oxygen just as hydrogen peroxide does. It should thus become obvious that anything bad said about the nascent (free radical) oxygen released by hydrogen peroxide also is equally true about chlorine peroxide.

If you doubt my word about whether you have chlorine dioxide when you buy one of these 'oxygen donor' products, just put a few drops on your forefinger and rub your thumb over it a few times. The unmistakable odor of chlorine (everyone recognizes Clorox) is present and stays with you for some time. I know some are going to swear that they do not have chlorine dioxide in their formulations. OK, if it isn't chlorine dioxide, it will be one of the close chemical cousins also containing chlorine. By the simple & revealing smell test, you will soon know. Here are the chemical bondings of some of the possible oxygen-containing products which can be used:

    H-O-Cl-O ($HClO_2$)   Chlorous Acid
    Na-O-Cl-O ($NaClO_2$)   Sodium Chlorite
    O-Cl-O (ClO_2)   Chlorine Dioxide

All of these compounds leave chlorine as a waste product of the breakdown; not necessarily a toxic amount, but enough that I have chosen non-chlorine-containing, oxygen-bearing compounds as my products of choice. Chlorine dioxide is made from sodium chlorate, sulfuric acid and methanol or from sodium chlorate and sulfur dioxide. When it breaks down, chlorine is left as a residual in the body and many health-conscious individuals are aware that chlorine has been associated with both cancer and heart disease.

One of the most absurd misstatements made about hydrogen peroxide is that it will induce, or increase the severity of Candidiasis & EBV (Chronic Fatigue Syndrome). One of these is caused by an overgrowth of a yeast-turned-fungus, the other is associated with a virus. Can water and oxygen (the component parts of hydrogen peroxide) cause either a virus or a fungus? Come on folks, let's stay within rational limits when we write our articles. The fact is both Candidiasis and Chronic Fatigue Syndrome are very responsive to the use of hydrogen peroxide and thousands of individuals have had fantastic results using it.

My conclusion is very simple. Whatever the oxygen-containing compound used, you are going to get free radical (nascent or singlet) oxygen which will almost immediately combine with another free radical (nascent, singlet) oxygen to form a stable substance which we know as oxygen and is symbolized by O_2. You can choose the one you wish. They will all benefit you to some extent in my opinion. I choose to use hydrogen peroxide for infusion purposes and external use and a combination of hydrogen peroxide and magnesium peroxide for oral ingestion for the following reasons:

1) Hydrogen peroxide is the richest and purest source of oxygen of any of these substances, thus it is ideal for use in intravenous solutions.
2) Hydrogen peroxide has a long and illustrious history of use as an external disinfectant for oral hygiene, etc. Thus for nasal spray use, mouth wash, tooth gel and other external uses, it still remains the product of choice.
3) Magnesium peroxide is less controversial for oral ingestion and does not have the obnoxious taste that hydrogen peroxide does. It is even more stable than the other oxygen containing compounds so it makes an ideal partner for hydrogen peroxide for internal use.

It is my hope that this will clarify in your mind the choices you have in liquid oxygen-containing products and allow you to make an intelligent decision without being misled. Knowledge and understanding will keep you from being confused by advertising hype.

Table of Contents

Miracle Oxygen	10
Father Wilhelm & Wally Grotz	11
Free Radical Flap	13
Who's Behind the Tree	15
The Secret - Oxygen	16
A Study of Rheumatoid Arthritis	19
The Elements of Life	23
Factors Causing Oxygen Depletion	26
Oxygen Impact on Health	31
Oxidation of Toxins	33
Candidiasis	34
Arthritis	37
Cancer	39
EBV and other Viral Disorders	40
Using Hydrogen Peroxide	42
Oral Ingestion	44
Bathing, Douches, Enemas, Etc	46
Obtaining 35% Food Grade H_2O_2	50
Hydrogen Peroxide in Agriculture	52
Ozone	63
Ozone or Hydrogen Peroxide?	66
Summary	67
Bibliography	69

Miracle Oxygen

The recent explosion of interest in the oral and infusion use of hydrogen peroxide heralds one of the greatest advances in the treatment of ailments of mankind in recent history. The impact this will have on future generations is almost impossible to imagine. This simple substance, known for decades, has the ability to change the course of human suffering by releasing cleansing and purifying oxygen to the body. Because one must truly understand the role of oxygen in living tissue, I will spend some time in elaborating on its many functions.

But don't think that I embraced hydrogen peroxide with open arms. Quite the opposite! I had always answered those who asked me about hydrogen peroxide with a negative response, indicating that peroxides were "free radicals" and certainly not something that one would want to contaminate his or her body with. After all, I had pretty much accepted the free radical concept of chronic degenerative disease, and like so many others (professional & lay person alike) considered peroxide a nasty instigator of problems.

My eventual interest to investigate this substance came from an unusual source, my wife. Although she is a faithful listener to my lectures and has heard me condemn hydrogen peroxide many times, she took the time to listen to Wally Grotz and Father Wilhelm expound on the benefits of hydrogen peroxide. Since I thought I had much better things to do than listen to a retired postmaster and a retired priest talk about health, I had never really heard the story. My wife indicated she was going to start taking peroxide and requested that I please find out as much as I could about it.

After this terrible blow to my ego, I decided that I would get the research data which would convince my wife of the terrors of hydrogen peroxide. What a time I had when the first pile of research was sent to me and I began to absorb the simple truth of a product which works on such a basic level that it is almost too good to be true. I transformed from a peroxide negative to a peroxide enthusiast in a short time. It shouldn't have come as too much of a surprise. My life has been a combination of rerouting erroneous beliefs and of rediscovering the work of others which has never been exposed, but instead gathered dust in library archives.

Father Wilhelm and Wally Grotz

The story of Father Wilhelm, who was a good friend of a Dr. Rosenow of the Mayo Clinic, is enthralling. Dr. Rosenow was a fine doctor, but an even greater researcher. His contention that many of the ills of mankind were the result of microbial contamination in a defense-poor body has never been challenged. He further contended that certain microbes were resistant to most of the medicines of man and attempted to find a substance which would destroy such organisms. His answer in the form of hydrogen peroxide came late in life and he died before ever seeing his discovery made public knowledge.

Father Wilhelm, besides being a friend of Dr Rosenow, was also a chemistry teacher and thus had an interest in the work Rosenow was pursuing. One of his attempts to further the discovery of the beneficial aspects of hydrogen peroxide was to present research to various pharmaceutical companies, feeling they could benefit from the findings and market products to the public. The answer was always the same, "Very nice, but no commercial value. It can't be patented, and it is very inexpensive. We're not interested."

Walter Grotz, retired postmaster, also has a great human interest story. Shortly after retirement, Mrs. Grotz convinced Wally they should go on a cruise to the Caribbean Islands, something they had always wanted to do, but never had the time. Wally had been suffering with arthritis for some time and really wanted to just putter around the house but, as good husbands often do, acceded to his wife's wishes and went on the trip. The chaplain on the cruise ship was none other than our aforementioned Father Wilhelm who, when he learned that Wally had arthritis, began preaching his "peroxide sermon." To make a long story short, Wally began taking hydrogen peroxide (H_2O_2) and was totally relieved of his arthritis in several weeks. He became as strongly motivated as Father Wilhelm and has literally dedicated his life to disseminating the truth about hydrogen peroxide. I take great pride in calling both these humanitarians friends and will always be grateful for their unselfish work.

The Free Radical Flap

The most misunderstood aspect of hydrogen peroxide is the contention that it is a free radical. This is simply not true! First of all, let's define a free radical. It is an element or compound which has an unpaired or unmatched electron. This lack of balance causes this substance to have a very reactive character. However, it must be noted that these free radicals are very short lived - usually in the one ten-thousandth of a second range. But during this short time, these free radicals can cause damage by joining with other body chemicals and changing their character, sometimes even producing a chain reaction by creating new free radicals that carry on.

That is the bad side. There is also a good side to free radicals, but let us see what happens to hydrogen peroxide when it first enters the body through the blood stream which could be from oral ingestion or by infusion.

$$\text{Hydrogen Peroxide} + \text{Catalase} = \text{Water} + O$$

When hydrogen peroxide enters the blood stream, an enzyme which is very prevalent in the human body almost immediately breaks it down to water and atomic oxygen, also called singlet oxygen or free radical oxygen.

$$O + O = O_2$$

Again in less than one ten-thousandth of a second, the atomic oxygen has become stable O_2 oxygen by pairing with another atomic oxygen. O_2 is the kind of oxygen the human body uses all the time. There is no time for the unstable atomic oxygen to get to a cell and cause any damage.

As mentioned before, there are beneficial free radicals, and one of them happens to be the atomic oxygen released when hydrogen peroxide is formed in the white blood cell (leukocyte) known as a macrophage which has a special area called a peroxisome which produces hydrogen peroxide. This is broken down to water and atomic (reactive or free radical) oxygen which will literally kill an invading bacteria allowing the macrophage to engulf and destroy the harmful organism.

Another example of free radical benefit is carbon monoxide (CO), a deadly form of gas which can kill the human organism if inhaled in large enough quantities. It can be inhaled but not exhaled, thus it piles up in the blood stream reducing the amount of stable oxygen which can be carried to the cells where it is needed. In order to decrease the amount of carbon monoxide in the blood stream, it must be changed to carbon dioxide (CO_2) a form of gas which is readily exhaled. This is accomplished by the simple mechanism of adding a singlet oxygen to the carbon monoxide. As with all good things, there are good characteristics to free radicals as well as bad.

Who's Behind the Tree?

The most vociferous of those who condemn hydrogen peroxide has written a book on the subject of reactive oxygens. In an attempt to overwhelm the reader with scientific references, the writer has filled the pages with sentences taken out of context, and used innuendo and theoretical assumptions to "prove" a point, namely that hydrogen peroxide is in some way harmful to the body. I am always first to welcome controversy, because I believe that out of controversy comes truth. But you don't try to pull the wool over someone's eyes by contorting and interpreting research in a slanted fashion.

It is interesting to note that this same individual is promoting the sale of another oxygen free radical-releasing substance - chlorine dioxide - also known as chlorine peroxide. The name should tell you something; it is made up of chlorine and oxygen. There is a nagging question in my mind as to why one would condemn one substance that offers singlet or atomic oxygen and praise another which in fact offers the same oxygen but leaves a toxic waste product in the body. Let's compare the two...

    Chlorine Dioxide $50.00/pint   47% Oxygen
    Hydrogen Peroxide $10.00/pint   94% Oxygen

The facts are that hydrogen peroxide is a better buy and contains twice as much oxygen per volume as does chlorine dioxide. Magnesium peroxide also provides an excellent source of oxygen in a very palatable form. But you can make up your own mind as to which to use, all will give up oxygen.

The Secret - Oxygen

In order to understand the marvelous things that the peroxides are capable of you really need to know all about oxygen, the substance which is formed when peroxide is cleaved by the enzyme, catalase.

We think of contaminated air as being laden with toxic substances which can damage us but often overlook the fact that as these substances contaminate the air, they also replace oxygen. In so doing, they may leave us with suboptimum amounts of oxygen as we breathe which may produce some serious consequences, such as an inability to concentrate, a sense of fatigue, an inability to repair and rejuvenate cells, etc.

The response of the ailing, especially the arthritic, to various atmospheric conditions is Nature's clue to the cause of degenerative disease. The unhealthfulness of a damp climate and the converse remedial benefit of a dry climate are frequent topics of conversation. The increase in aches and pains of some arthritics before a storm is a matter of common knowledge. Even the most vigorous are sometimes affected by atmospheric changes. This is because of a decrease of oxygen in the atmosphere under certain conditions.

There are two reasons for a decrease of oxygen in the air we inhale...

1) Molecules of moisture displace a portion of the oxygen.
2) Low barometric pressure resulting in fewer molecules of oxygen per cubic inch of space.

Either condition results in less oxygen in the air we inhale.

Both molecules of oxygen and molecules of moisture are invisible spheres occupying space. An atmosphere in which molecules of moisture are mixed with molecules of oxygen contains less oxygen than one in which there are fewer molecules of moisture, such as in a comparatively dry atmosphere. This can be compared by considering two baskets of fruit; one being a mixture of apples and oranges, the other containing only apples. Obviously there are fewer apples in the basket in which oranges are intermingled than in the one containing only apples, even as there is less oxygen in a breath inhaled in which there is considerable moisture.

The factor of low atmospheric pressure adds to the lack of oxygen in the air inhaled. In order to make this perfectly clear, let us consider two extremes...

1) The air pressure in a tire forces the molecules in the tire closer together.
2) Conversely, the low pressure on a mountain top allows the molecules to spread farther apart.

One says "The air is thin." Thus we see that low pressure reduces the proportion of oxygen in the air inhaled.

Another negative factor is the lessened efficiency of the elimination of the poisonous gases in the lungs. As a damp dish towel is less efficient in absorbing moisture than a dry towel, so damp air is less efficient in absorbing the most toxin-laden gas from the lungs.

Thus we find three factors - a damp atmosphere, low barometric pressure and inefficient elimination subtracting from the vitalizing effect of a more favorable atmosphere. Ideally a high margin of oxygen molecules float in the blood stream, ready, eager and able to trigger the processes of life.

The ailing, more noticeably the arthritic, often suffer when they are unable to extract enough oxygen from the air they breathe. This justifies the suspicion that there is a lack of oxygen in the blood stream with a possible high toxin level. This high toxin level can be reduced by an increase in the amount of oxygen in the blood stream. Perhaps you have observed the action of hydrogen peroxide on an infected wound. The oxygen attacks the infected matter in boiling fury. While there is not this extreme reaction in the blood stream, bacteria cannot live in an environment in which there is a dominant proportion of oxygen. As oxygen is required to cleanse antagonistic matter from the blood stream, we can again suspect a low level of oxygen and a high toxin level in those who show evidence of lowered vitality.

A Study of Rheumatoid Arthritis

Dr Bernard Edstrom brought conclusive facts and figures to light, furnishing concrete proof of low oxygen levels. The report, in essence, was as follows.

He constructed a simulated dry tropical climate in the wing of a hospital near Lund, Sweden. The air was kept very dry and a temperature of 89.6 degrees F was maintained. A half-and-half mixture of rheumatic fever and rheumatoid arthritic patients was admitted.

Rheumatoid arthritis is the type in which the muscular tissues are contracted, depriving them of the flexibility required for normal mobility. It is also called rheumatism. Certain blood tests were made before admittance and the major abnormalities noted were...

1) The sedimentation rate in the blood was very high.
2) The blood was a dark, unhealthy hue.
3) The oxygen saturation of the blood in the veins was a very low average of 52%.

Imagine this group as they entered with canes or on crutches. Their misery caused many of them to be very disagreeable. Marital discord was common among them. As they settled in their new quarters, many noted changes in their bodies. They began to move with greater ease in a very short time. Wives began to receive love letters. They reported feeling happier and more optimistic.

At the end of one hundred days, blood tests were again taken. These are some of the findings...

1) The sedimentation rate was greatly reduced.
2) The dark, unhealthy hue of the blood was replaced by the red color physicians have noted in primitive people in various areas who are free from degenerative disease. This red color indicates a high oxygen level. This has been noted in Eskimos, Hunzas, natives of the hinterland of Australia and some tribes of Africa. Degenerative diseases are almost unknown to them.
3) The oxygen saturation of the blood in the veins had risen from 52% to an extremely satisfactory 82%.
4) The bacteria found in the throats of the rheumatic fever patients had disappeared.

The disappearance of the bacteria was because these organisms cannot live in an atmosphere dominated by oxygen. Apparently the most significant point was overlooked in this study: *The bacteria would have been destroyed upon invasion of the body had there been an abundance of oxygen present. Thus no bodily damage from their presence could have taken place. Also, oxygen dissolved the sediment. Here again, the presence of adequate oxygen would have barred the formation of this sediment in the first place.*

Such sediment not only obstructs the circulation of the blood, but also accumulates to form concretions in the gallbladder, kidneys, heart, arterial walls, eyes, etc. For a moment, consider the 52% oxygen blood from the veins entering the liver. Most of the oxygen in this inferior blood is bound up in the molecules of proteins, carbohydrates, fats, water and carbon dioxide. The only oxygen available is furnished from the arteries. The liver's burden of sanitation is very heavy due to excess toxins in such blood. There is a lack of oxygen necessary to inspire the enzymes in their various performances of the many processes necessary in the liver.

The Result: The liver produces an inferior substance to nourish the cells resulting in poor regeneration, rejuvenation and restoration of cells.

The 82% oxygenated blood entering the liver presents a very encouraging aspect. Probably 30% of this oxygen is free molecules not involved with any other element. The burden of sanitation is light because blood with a goodly supply of oxygen is quite free of toxins. There is also a bountiful supply of oxygen to inspire the enzymes to their greatest efficiency.

The Result: A superior nutrient mix is now available to nourish the cells resulting in vigorous regeneration, rejuvenation and restoration of cells.

This contention of mine, that a dominating proportion of oxygen is a barrier to all degenerative diseases, is based on sound reasoning...

1) As stated previously, physicians have noted the bright red color of blood in the veins of various native peoples, denoting a high oxygen saturation.
2) Physicians have also noted these same peoples' immunity to most, if not all, the degenerative diseases that civilized man suffers from.
3) At Hospital Santa Monica in Rosarito Beach, Baja California, Mexico and Institut Santa Monica in KamienPomorsky, Poland, we routinely see the blood of patients change color as they improve in their health.
4) It is a well-established and accepted fact that the darker the blood color, the less oxygen it carries and the brighter red its color, the more oxygen present.

> *Donsbach's Theory: The degree of the vitality of the body and the strength of the barrier to degenerative diseases is in proportion to the ratio of oxygen's saturation of the blood stream, all things being equal.*

The Elements of Life

The four major elements generating life are as follows...

    nitrogen + carbon + hydrogen + oxygen = **protein**
    carbon + hydrogen + oxygen = **carbohydrates**
    hydrogen + oxygen = **water**
    oxygen + carbohydrates = **energy**

These constitute the major substances in the blood stream. The minor elements are not of present concern. Nitrogen, hydrogen and oxygen are mildly magnetic. The conventional terms "negative" and "positive" polarity are confusing; therefore, the terms I use are...

Active Polarity	Counterative Polarity	Neutral
Oxygen	Hydrogen	Carbon
Nitrogen		

Metabolism = Anabolism + Catabolism

The processes of animal life fall into the classifications anabolism and catabolism. Metabolism refers to the sum of both.

    Oxygen is catabolic
    Hydrogen is anabolic

Since catabolism is essentially the breaking down of tissue into simpler and easier to dispose of substances, oxygen dissolves, disintegrates and deconcentrates substances.

Anabolism is the building up of tissue, so hydrogen solidifies, integrates and concentrates substances.

The food processor takes advantage of the concentrating properties of hydrogen. He forces it into vegetable oil, concentrating it into solid vegetable shortening and margarine. In so doing, he also creates what are called "trans-fatty acids" which the body is incapable of breaking down. (A little tip - never eat margarine - it is a bad food.)

Since metabolism is the sum total of anabolism and catabolism, we could sum the process up like this...

Anabolism maintains the stable form of the body. Catabolism maintains the mobility of the body.

Hydrogen concentrates the proteins which compose the building blocks that create the stable form of the cell. Oxygen reduces the old, used-up, tired cellular tissue to easily eliminated substances to prevent fixation.

When oxygen levels fall in the internal environment of man, the housecleaning functions requlnng oxygen are diminished. Such lack of function is termed *congestion* when found in animal life; ie, liver, lung, heart, muscular, etc. This congestion can also involve the circulatory system.

The average oxygen saturation of the veins in modern man ranges from 60 to 70%. This is too low! Fifty-two percent oxygen saturation, is perhaps the lowest level which can sustain life. Cleansing the blood stream of toxins and building up the oxygen level can be compared to cleaning the ashes and clinkers from the furnace and opening the draft, transforming a smoky, smoldering fire into a clean, brilliant flame. The transformation which can take place in the body is fantastic.

Perhaps you have felt a warm, exhilarating glow after building up the oxygen level through brisk exercise accompanied by deep and rapid breathing. This is but a hint of the delightful results of decongestion through the oxidation reduction system which our body uses to detoxify itself.

In the presence of 82% oxygen saturation, which we talked about, there is a dramatic increase in energy and a change for the better in our nervous system. Irritability and nervousness vanish. Obviously, oxygen must dominate over the stabilizing hydrogen in order for the mobility of the body to be sustained. Have you ever wondered why you don't want to move when you are ill?

Factors Causing Oxygen Depletion

Many factors are involved in causing oxygen depletion. One of the most overlooked is the fact that a few hundred years ago the oxygen content of our atmosphere was about 35% - today it is about 19%. We have had an almost 50% decrease in the available oxygen in the air around us!

Mineral deficiencies are another factor. Minerals have been overshadowed by the publicity given vitamins, despite the fact that minerals are actually more critical to the life process. Many minerals are active in the prevention of the formation of hydrogenated toxins. Their deficiency increases the burden of detoxification upon oxygen, exhausting it at a more rapid pace. Dr. Decoty-Marsh of England reports great success in treating arthritis through the administration of potassium. This mineral is king in its capacity for inhibiting the formation of toxins.

Copper is involved in the assimilation of calcium, phosphorus and iron. A copper deficiency is serious. An iron deficiency in the blood stream also reduces its oxygen-carrying capacity. Cobalt and vitamins B-1 and B-12 also aid in the assimilation of iron in the blood. This is an example of the importance of the combination of both minerals and vitamins.

In the absence of oxygen to counteract excess waste acids in the stomach, calcium unites with other substances to form calcium hydroxide, a useless and potentially harmful substance that also binds the calcium so that it cannot be absorbed into the blood stream.

Cattle suffer from mineral deficiencies. Several herds in northern California developed a form of arthritis. It was found that the ground upon which they grazed was deficient in phosphorus. Phosphoric acid was injected hypodermically or mixed with their feed. The ground on which they grazed was fertilized with phosphorus. The cattle were cured. This places the statement made freely by the FDA that there is no difference in the quality of plants regardless of characteristics of the soil in a very questionable position.

The Hunzas are noted for their long life and vigor. They irrigate their farms with the mineralized water from the melting snow on the mountain tops. They also take advantage of every particle of organic fertilizer. Across the stream running through the Hunza valley are a far less vigorous, shorter-lived people. It was found that their farms were very deficient in minerals, perhaps accounting for their lack of vitality.

Certain authorities, such as the FDA, contradict the Department of Agriculture by stating that the nutritional qualities of a plant do not vary - that crops grown on well-fertilized ground may vary from crops grown on poor soil in quantity but not in quality.

My observations contradict this. A neighbor planted potatoes on ground, part of which had been planted in alfalfa the year before, which leaves nutrient-dense soil. Most insects detest plants raised on well-fertilized soil. They stripped the plants right up to the previous alfalfa ground, but did not touch the more luxuriant growth on the richer soil. This little incident tends to prove the fallacy of the authorities' aforesaid opinion. But, of course, these authorities are not always interested in facts.

The lack of minerals throws an extra burden on oxygen.

1) A lack of minerals detracts from the body's manufacture of digestive and other enzymes. Poor digestion leaves undigested substances to form antagonistic debris that oxygen must cleanse from the body.
2) A lack of minerals promotes the formation of toxins, increasing the need for more oxygen.
3) A lack of certain minerals induces anemia, lessening the ability of the blood to carry oxygen.

Overeating can also cause a real oxygen deficiency. Not only is more oxygen required to complete the digestive process but because of the excess of food, there is also an excess of toxic metabolic waste products that must be dealt with. Ever wonder why you feel so tired after a big meal?

Improper breathing techniques can also deplete the amount of oxygen you should have to really function well. Deep breathing exercises indulged in for 3 to 5 minutes every day help to train you to breathe properly all the time. Remember that proper breathing comes from the diaphragm and not the shoulders. The chest and lower abdomen should expand when breathing correctly.

Negative mental attitudes can become a major factor in oxygen depletion. Think for a moment, perhaps you remember the last time you felt depressed. Were you breathing in a shallow fashion? In addition, the very thought patterns that are associated with negativity and depression produce toxins in the body that increase the need for detoxifying oxygen. Consider the use of meditative techniques, the power of positive thinking, subliminal suggestion or any other means of making you feel positive and happy.

Any infective process, chronic or acute, places a great strain on the oxygen reserve because of the toxins associated with the infection. Never overlook a chronic infection however small it may be. Infected teeth are a great contributor to many diseases because they decrease the body's ability to defend itself.

Another contributor to oxygen depletion which is often unnoticed is the use of fluoride in our drinking water. The *Spotlight* newspaper wrote on February 4, 1985, "Recently, Russian investigators have found that fluoride, which is being added to drinking water, slows down the process of burning food (called oxidation) and lowers the level of adenosine triphosphate (ATP). When the body bums food, it stores the energy in a substance called ATP During fluoride intoxication it is reported that rats and mice have a decreased oxygen uptake, reduced expiration of air, and decreased activity of the oxidation reduction enzymes in the liver and lungs. By the third month of use, 31 to 40% decreases in ATP levels were observed in all organs. Differences in the response of red blood cells, liver, muscle, and brain to the fluorosis were observed after 30 days of use." (Note: Fluoride has just been linked to bone cancer in addition to all its other negative properties. We must stop drinking this toxin and stop using it as an additive to toothpastes, rinses, etc. It is illegal to use any product that causes cancer in our food or water supply!)

Most of the reasons for oxygen depletion in your body can be averted by common sense procedures. However, there may come a time when you wish to enhance the oxygen content in your blood stream. That is when you might wish to consider the use of a drink made of magesium peroxide which not only tastes good but which generally makes people feel much better, even if they didn't feel bad when they started taking it.

Oxygen Impact on Health

You should now appreciate the tremendous impact oxygen has on your health and well-being. The addition of small amounts of oxygen to the blood stream can have tremendous effect. As early as 1904, physicians were trying oxygen infusions in dying patients and noting results. In 1940, two doctors treated several patients with severe pulmonary disease with oxygen infusions and reported that all patients improved.

The use of infused hydrogen peroxide was reported in 1920 during the influenza epidemic. Although excellent response was noted, there was no follow-up and the concept of hydrogen peroxide infusions was allowed to languish, to the best of my knowledge, until I began experimenting with it in early 1985. I have found that some research was done at Baylor University using hydrogen peroxide intra-arterially in conjunction with radiation therapy for cancer. Here again, the results were favorable but it certainly didn't receive any press, nor were doctors in general notified.

I was quite enthused when I started, primarily because I felt that this was the perfect answer for Systemic Candidiasis, a condition which has resisted th best drugs and diets ever devised. My biggest problems was in determining the amount to use on an individual because there was little research as to the amount that would be tolerated by a patient. More important was how much should be used in the treatment of various specific disorders. How much was too much?

Using myself as a guinea pig, I had the doctors who work with me at Hospital Santa Monica stand around me with emergency equipment on the ready and proceeded to inject myself with a diluted solution of 35% food grade hydrogen peroxide. What a white-knuckle few minutes! But there were no emboli (bubbles in the blood stream which could cause serious or even fatal problems), and the only changes I felt were a slight warming sensation and a feeling of clearness in my head. Using this as a basis, I slowly began infusing patients with this solution. I found that dimethylsulfoxide (DMSO) was a catalyst and produced better results, but other substances could cause a premature oxidative reaction that produced pain and discomfort, as well as decreasing the effectiveness. Between Hospital Santa Monica and Institut Santa Monica, we have now administered over 30,000 infusions of hydrogen peroxide without a single problem. I am positive in my mind that this methodology is a safe and effective tool in the treatment of a wide diversity of illnesses.

Oxidation of Toxins

It should be emphasized here that the primary function of the intravenous use of hydrogen peroxide is the increase of oxygen available to do its job of housecleaning. By oxidizing toxins, a great load is taken off all systems in the body and functions return to normal in a short period of time. It is this rapid reversal of symptoms that is so difficult to explain to a candidiasis patient who has had sensitivities to every food under the sun, but in five days are eating foods that have been prohibited for years. They are so used to living a cloistered life and denying themselves everything that when we serve buckwheat pancakes (as we do once a week at the hospital) they are shocked. It doesn't seem possible that pancakes (of any kind) can be eaten with impunity.

You must understand that the oxidation reduction system the body uses to get rid of toxins will often remove the very things that were making you sensitive (allergic). It is the most efficient and well-designed detoxification for the human body possible. Colonies, fasts, herbal cleansers, etc, all pale to insignificance before this system. And all that is needed is adequate oxygen.

May I please encourage you to learn more about this if you have any further questions or doubts. Healing comes from within and anything we can do to enhance such is positive. The use of drugs which are known poisons will never be the answer to the ills of mankind.

Candidiasis

The use of hydrogen peroxide in the treatment of candidiasis was one of the first applications I devised for this wonderful oxygen donor. A condition popularized by Drs Truss and Crook with their books on the subject of candidiasis was long thought of as a condition primarily for women, and then usually only of the vaginal tract area. It also frequently occurs in the mouths of children as *thrush* and is often associated with advanced illnesses of all kinds.

The commonly accepted concept as to the migration of the organism *candida albicans* from the intestinal tract where it is normally present, to the internal environment of the body, is based on the overuse of antibiotic medications, the use of steroid hormones such as cortisone and birth control pills. Obviously the antibiotics will destroy the natural bacterial flora which abound in the intestinal tract and literally eat the candida, keeping it under control. When they are destroyed by antibiotics, the yeast can multiply explosively.

This does not explain the migration from the gut to internal environments of the body. Such could be the result of a weak or damaged gut membrane that would allow the candida to travel into the blood stream throughout the body. But the use of the substances mentioned does explain why so many females suffer from chronic candidiasis since the overgrowth of the yeast in the gut will eventually migrate to the vaginal tract and set up residence there in a warm, moist environment that it likes so well.

The common treatment for candidiasis has been the use of *Nystatin*, an antifungal used for a variety of yeasts and fungi. Unfortunately, it has failed for many. *Nystatin* is primarily effective because it is poorly absorbed through the gut wall and thus remains in the gut and can effectively control a yeast overgrowth in that area. It can also be applied as an ointment or cream in the vaginal area or as a suppository.

All this is well and good, but what about the unfortunate individual who has the problem in the internal areas of the body, known as <u>Systemic Candidiasis</u>? It just doesn't work! Some doctors use *Ketoconazole*, a liver-toxic drug (Note the following warning in the Physician's Desk Reference: "*Ketoconazole has been associated with hepatic toxicity, **including some fatalities**. Patients receiving this drug should be informed by the physician of the risk and should be closely monitored*").

Ketoconazole is effective for some cases of Systemic Candidiasis, but I have seen many patients who had serious problems still remaining following as much as six months' use, which is excessive. Normally it should not be given for more than thirty days.

There is a plethora of wholistic approaches to candidiasis available. These include caprylic acid, garlic, various herbs, etc. Then there are the rigid diets that want to blame foods that contain sugar and yeast as the cause of the problem. That simply is not true. It is true that these foods may aggravate the condition, but they do not cause it. If these diets and approaches were successful in controlling or eliminating candidiasis, it would not continue to be a problem.

Many hundreds of sufferers have called me and said "I've done it all and I still have a problem. The MD's with their medicine only made me sicker and the natural things may have helped me a bit, but I still have my problem." Here is where I began gingerly using hydrogen peroxide, both orally and intravenously. First we started with the oral formulation and found that more than half of those with symptoms were able to respond very favorably. But there was still a large group who were not doing well.

So I began infusing these 'problem' patients with a dilute solution of 35% food grade hydrogen peroxide. The results were outstanding! I did find out that I had to have at least 19 to 21 days to clean the body of the fungus. Anything less was not enough and for a few, we even had to go twenty-eight days.

It should thus become very apparent that the proper way to approach the condition of candidiasis, particularly intestinal, is the use of oral oxygen in the form of magnesium peroxide. If this is not effective, then you should consider going to a doctor who uses hydrogen peroxide intravenously. I know there area few in the United States, but don't count on them to last long. My experience with the FDA and other governmental agencies is that they quickly snuff out alternative therapies that work too well.

Arthritis

My first contact with a real live arthritis sufferer who had recovered through the use of hydrogen peroxide was Walter Grotz, a retired postmaster from Delano, Minnesota. If there is anyone who is less likely to respond to the placebo effect than a postmaster, I would like to meet them. Walter convinced me (after his lovely wife verified it) that he had recovered from a very painful and motion-limiting arthritis in a period of six weeks after beginning the use of oral hydrogen peroxide. Since then I have talked to dozens of recovered arthritics, some who drank it, some who bathed in it and drank it and some who only bathed in it.

If you have known anyone who has arthritis, or if you have it yourself, you will know that the pain relievers, the non-steroidal anti-inflammatories and other medications are only temporary relief at best. The vast majority of sufferers have been told so many times that there really isn't anything that can be done for them that they believe it themselves. When something does cause a change it is very noticable.

We know it is oxygen which does the work of normalizing the joints in arthritis. Most of the research up to this point has been done with hydrogen peroxide, so the standards regulating the amounts one would take are based upon a specific number of drops of 35% food grade hydrogen peroxide. Thus the label of a product might say "Each tablespoonful contains the amount of oxygen as found in (10) or (20) drops of 35% food grade hydrogen peroxide." This is for reference only and creates a standard for comparison.

It has been my experience that in order for results to be obtained, the equivalent effective dose is equal to a minimum of 75 drops of 35% food grade hydrogen peroxide daily. This will most often require the intake of approximately four ounces of a magnesium peroxide solution, which is the form I now use orally.

Please understand that there are serious problems which can result from the mishandling of the 35% food grade hydrogen peroxide which is the reason that for the past several years I have always cautioned those interested to not have it stored in their home except under very rigid circumstances. The ultimate negative occurred when a family had a bottle of 35% food grade hydrogen peroxide stored in their refrigerator. A neighbor boy, mistaking it for water, drank some straight and immediately began vomiting. He inhaled some of the vomitus and died from suffocation. This is the only case of death that I know of, but it is certainly reason enough for one to rationally choose the magnesium peroxide alternative.

AN IMPORTANT RULE TO REMEMBER: Whichever solution you take, it is best used on an empty stomach in order to avoid oxidation which then leaves nothing for the blood stream and very little, if any, effect on whatever you are trying to help your body accomplish.

Cancer

The award-winning work of Dr. Otto Warburg, a Nobel Prize winner, led us to the knowledge that the cancer cell is primarily anaerobic, just like most bacteria. The presence of increased amounts of oxygen will inhibit the spread of cancer cells and will eventually cause them to die. The obvious step was to infuse cancer patients with hydrogen peroxide and see if there was any unusual progress noted.

We found immediately that many cancer patients were aware of a sensation of heat in the area of the cancer, often during the infusion. Sometimes this was unpleasant, but more often it was merely a warming sensation. In some "close to the surface" tumors such as might be found in breast cancer, we often observe an erythematous (red) patch appearing on the skin.

I have been so impressed with the results of the use of hydrogen peroxide that every cancer patient receives infusions of the 35% food grade hydrogen peroxide/ DMSO mixture throughout their entire stay. Many of our patients come specifically for this treatment although I use other medications such as thymosin, interferon, cesium chloride, carbamide, hydrazine sulfate, isoprinosin, laetrile, clodronate, mistletoe, oncotox, levamisol, EFA Forte and others depending on the type of cancer and the condition of the patient. But it should be apparent where I rank hydrogen peroxide, since this is the only substance I use in EVERY cancer patient.

EBV and Other Viral Disorders

Epstein Barr Virus (EBV) is associated with a condition now called Chronic Fatigue Syndrome. It is characterized by an overwhelming feeling of fatigue and aches and pains such as one would normally associate with the flu, as well as a mental change which usually leaves one in a constant state of depression. It has only recently become the object of some rather intense scrutiny. Prior to this it was generally thought of as a hypochondriac's paradise because there were no acute symptoms associated with it.

Wholistic physicians were criticized for diagnosing and treating it because it was just not recognized as a disease entity. Now that offical support groups have been formed, many researchers have documented its existence and although general confusion reigns as to why it occurs, we at least have proof that it exists.

There are other viral conditions which produce similar symptoms, cytomegalo virus being one. All these conditions have one thing in common - the protective immune system of the individual is not working up to par. In the case of EBV, the virus associated with mononucleosis apparently lies dormant in the body for some time before it decides to surface and cause problems. But as with all such viral-related disorders, it seems to be very picky as to whom it chooses as its victim. Certainly not everyone who had mononucleosis is going to be a victim of the Chronic Fatigue Syndrome; no more than all those who had the chicken pox as a child will get shingles as an adult (shingles is associated with the chicken pox virus, of the herpes family which lies dormant in the nerves, sometimes to erupt with a fierce outbreak).

Our approach to these viral conditions at the two hospitals is to use one of the best antivirals I know of - isoprinosin - to slow down the viral replication. Any of the viral conditions utilize the DNA of the cell to produce replication. One virus invading the cell will produce thousands of new viruses which go on to repeat the cycle. This is why we can truthfully refer to the "explosive multiplication" of viruses under the proper conditions.

The body has several defenses against viruses, one of which is the production of an impervious coat of armor which it will quickly fashion if in danger of invasion. Interferon seems to be the only catalyst for the production of this armor and therefore, the use of this expensive but valuable substance is often called for in viral-related conditions.

It has been our experience that most of the Chronic Fatigue Syndrome patients have very low glandular function, so we use live cell therapy with particular attention to the adrenals, thyroid and thymus.

All viruses are inhibited by a high oxygen environment. Used intravenously, hydrogen peroxide is our method of choice to increase the oxygen content of the internal environment of the body.

Using Hydrogen Peroxide

The most important thing to remember is the kind of hydrogen peroxide to use.

35% Food Grade Hydrogen Peroxide

This is the only kind of hydrogen peroxide which should be ingested orally or used intravenously (a 30% reagent grade is also acceptable where the 35% is not available) but you must never consider using it at anywhere near this concentration!

YOU MUST ALWAYS DILUTE 35% HYDROGEN PEROXIDE OR RISK SERIOUS PROBLEMS!

I am being very aggressive about this warning because of the tremendous interest in this substance by so many individuals, some of whom do not have the healthy respect that one should give this concentrated oxidant. Cases of children picking up an unlabeled bottle out of the refrigerator, thinking it is water because it looks just as clear and drinking it has led to some serious consequences! If you keep 35% undiluted hydrogen peroxide in your home, be sure to lock it up to avoid accidental, unwise use.

I must stress that I personally prefer magnesium dioxide for oral use.

The hydrogen peroxide which you find at your drug store counter is 3% concentration and is fine for external use, but contains preservatives and stabilizers which should not be ingested orally. Thus you can use this to add to your bath water (from one pint to one quart, depending on your need or desire) but should not attempt to drink it. And while we are on this subject, I would like to encourage you to try a bath in this oxygen-rich substance. It invigorates. It relieves pain. It stimulates your mind. It reduces stiffness and soreness like no other treatment. We give all our patients a whirlpool bath with the equivalent of one gallon of the 3% in it every other day. Some might like to do this early in the day because it can be very invigorating and you won't want to go to bed right afterward.

Use in Bathing

Use 6 fluid ounces of the 35% food grade hydrogen peroxide in a bathtub full of rather warm water. Be sure that the area you have problems with is fully immersed and soak for 20 minutes or more. I have seen joints that are stiff and sore relieved in just a few baths. Skin problems also respond to this form of use, including rashes, eczema, psoriasis, athletes foot, etc. NOTE: 6 fluid ounces of 35% hydrogen peroxide is equivalent to about 2 quarts of 3% which is easily bought in any drug or grocery store. If the 35% is not readily available, you can use the 3% with just as many benefits for bathing.

As a Douche

The tissues in the vaginal tract are quite sensitive, so be sure to use the proper dilution if you wish to prepare your own. I have to recommend that you consider the prepared douche solution which is readily available and pH balanced so that no irritation will occur. If you prepare your own, use no more than 15 drops in a douche bag. If you use the prepared solution, instructions for retaining the solution for best results are included. Many of the minor irritations of the vaginal tract as well as yeast infections will respond very well to this method.

Enemas

Never use the 35% in an Enema. There have been numerous incidences of individuals using several ounces of the 35% in an enema. This will almost always lead to bleeding and tissue damage in the rectum which will last for many, many days. Because of the high bacterial count in the lower bowel, heavy oxidation will occur when the peroxide is introduced. This can damage delicate mucous tissues as well as cause bleeding. Extreme caution should be exercised and if you wish to use it, do not use more than 15 drops per enema bag of water.

Use in the Kitchen

The oxidation reaction with bacteria makes hydrogen peroxide an ideal cleansing and purifying agent for fruits, vegetables, meats and fish. You can make your own wash by putting 4 ounces of 35% in a gallon of water. Passing your fruits and vegetables through this mixture before storing them in the refrigerator will increase their lifespan by several days. It will also remove all bacteria and most of the contaminants that may be on them. I prefer to spray this mixture on meats, chicken and fish. It does wonders to remove the odors from these foods and they seem to taste much better when cooked, probably because all bacteria are killed. A commercial spray is available which uses the extract of grapefruit seed which has bacteriocidal, virucidal and parasiticidal properties combined with hydrogen peroxide. It is truly a fine product!

Swimming Pools

The therapeutic pool at Hospital Santa Monica uses only hydrogen peroxide as a purifying agent. Our office has been inundated with calls from homeowners who want to use hydrogen peroxide in their swimming pools. It seems that many are now tired of the chlorine which is a known health hazard. The average pool will require about eight gallons to begin with, then adding from one-half to one gallon per week to maintain a 30 parts per million concentration. This can easily be measured by using test strips available from...

Lab Safety Supply
PO Box 1368
Janesville, WI 53437
(800) 356-0783

H_2O_2 Inc.
2560 Muhlenhardt Road
Shakopee, MN 55379
(612) 496-1417

Jerry Freeman
4853 Joyce Drive
Dayton, OH 45439
(513) 299-4283

You will have sparkling clear water, there will be no growth on the sides of the pool and, more important, you will not have red eyes from the irritation of the heavy amounts of chlorine in the pool water nor will your body be absorbing this dangerous chemical when you swim in it. NOTE: It has been estimated that full body contact for twenty minutes with chlorine-saturated water will allow absorption equivalent to drinking two quarts of the same water.

Home Gardening

Neither my wife or I have as much time as we would like to devote to growing things. However, my wife is quite faithful in tending her roses. She sprays them with a very dilute solution - 8 tablespoonfuls of *3%* hydrogen peroxide in a gallon of water - and has the finest roses in the neighborhood. You should also spray the ground at the base of your plants. Spray the same solution on cut flowers and add a little to the water to make them last 50% longer.

In Vaporizers

If you have a respiratory problem, use 12 ounces of the 3% hydrogen peroxide in one gallon of water in a cool mist vaporizer. It will be very beneficial in a wide variety of conditions such as emphysema, chronic obstructive pulmonary disease, bronchitis, pneumonia, etc.

Obtaining 35% Food Grade H_2O_2

35% food grade hydrogen peroxide is what got this show going. But I have to give a note of caution - not everyone gives this concentrated oxidizer the respect it deserves. If you store it in a warm place, gas will form and potentially cause a container to explode. If it is left out where others who do not know what it is, particularly in an unlabeled container, it can easily be mistaken for water. If consumed in an undiluted form, it can cause intense vomiting and if the vomitus is inhaled into the lungs, death can ensue.

For some unknown reason, individuals often use extremely high concentrations of this substance in douches and enemas. *I caution you: the maximum amount of the 35% hydrogen peroxide you should use in either instance should be measured in drops - approximately 15 drops in one quart of water - no more!* You will experience extreme discomfort and bleeding if you use too much.

For these reasons I recommend that individuals with small children refrain from having it around. For the rest of you, be sure that the container is certified to be a container for oxidants, that you store it in a cool, dark place and be careful when handling it so that you do not get it in your eyes.

35% food grade hydrogen peroxide is still available for use in water sterilization procedures, particularly as a replacement for chlorine in a swimming pool, so it may be purchased from most chemical houses in drums of 30 gallons or more. It is comparatively inexpensive in these quantities. Remember that it can cause your skin to whiten and sting for about twenty minutes after contact. Flush immediately with water if you do get some on your skin.

As I have said before, the 35% is not the best way to get therapeutic amounts into your blood stream because it tastes so bad that you cannot get enough into your stomach. It takes the equivalent of 80 to 150 drops per day in order to get to therapeutic levels. Thus my preference for magnesium dioxide-containing products.

Note: The following excerpt has been taken from ECH$_2$O$_2$, a publication authored by Walter Grotz, with permission. This address is PO Box 126, Delano, MN 55328. Mr. Grotz has the most complete file on hydrogen peroxide I know of. Thank you for your years of devotion to a humanitarian cause, Mr. Grotz.

Hydrogen Peroxide in Agriculture

MERCK'S INDEX indicates that hydrogen peroxide can be used as a water disinfectant. Always use 35% food grade hydrogen peroxide in a dilute solution. NEVER use it as a concentrate without diluting it first. To make a 3% solution, mix 1 ounce 35% food grade hydrogen peroxide with 11 ounces of water. Distilled water is best when feasible, especially if the solution is to be stored for any length of time.

The following information is for education purposes and is not meant to treat or prescribe. We are sharing what others have told us has worked for them as they seek to have healthier animals and plants. Man, too, will benefit further down the food chain.

It was in 1985 that the first dairy farmer began injecting hydrogen peroxide in the water system of his entire farm. The water on his farm was polluted and mastitis was a problem with this herd. After continual use since that time, this same farmer has noticed with satisfaction the healthy state of his cows. In April 1988, the butterfat content of his Holstein cows was up to 5.3%. Another farmer who weighs the milk from every cow at every milking reported that his milk production increased from 6 to 8 pounds per cow per milking. Others have reported their bacteria count has gone down to less than 2,000 per cubic centimeter. Many other farmers are continuing this experimental process.

For drinking water of farm animals use 8 ounces of 35% food grade hydrogen peroxide per 1,000 gallons of water, or 30 ppm. If you do not have an injector, start out by using 1 teaspoon of the 35% in the drinking cups at the stanchion. This same ratio is used for all farm animals: cows, pigs, poultry, sheep, goats, rabbits and birds, increasing the oxygen level to the blood and cells. When hydrogen peroxide has been used for cattle, an increase in milk production and butterfat content has been reported. Farmers have also reported less mastitis in their herds. Hog farmers have reported that they have been able to market their hogs using less feed in a shorter growing time (as much as 30 days less). Turkey and chicken growers reported increased weight per bird using less feed. A man in Wisconsin has told us that he has had the best reproduction rate of his buffalo by using hydrogen peroxide in their drinking water.

Peroxide application into the well water or city water can best be accomplished by a metering device which keeps the application more constant and thorough, although manual application can be a second best. The rule of thumb is 8 to

10 oz of 35% peroxide to 1,000 gallons of water in a holding tank or stock tank, striving to attain a reading of 30 ppm after application. In order to get a true reading of the amount of oxygen remaining in the water after the application, use Peroxide Test Strips designed especially for this very purpose.

When peroxide is being applied throughout the entire watering system, with a reading of 30 ppm at the end of the line, all the water should stay clean of rust, bacteria and algae, plus some other foreign materials found in some water. Thus the waterers stay clean and help to stop the spread of disease.

Through this method of water purification, we have seen cows pass worms, hogs in a hoghouse without even parasite eggs in the fecal matter (with no previous worming medication for an extended period of time) and some animals may cut back on feed, depending on the nutrient level in their feeding program. As long as the iron and mineral level in the body is where it should be, the peroxide will attract and hold oxygen in the blood and cells of the body allowing the body's fuel system to burn more efficiently. This process of water purification is especially helpful in a confinement barn of any animals.

In the dairy barn use as a pipeline rinse for milkstone. Depending on the length of the pipeline, as a rule, 2 to 4 ounces of 35% hydrogen peroxide to 15 gallons of water will work with good results. This amount also works for rinsing milk cans and the bulk tank to keep down bacteria as well as milkstone. (Note: If hydrogen peroxide is being injected into the water system at 30 ppm, the above ratio may need to be cut in half.)

For power wash in the dairy barn as well as the hog house in the sanitization process, mix enough peroxide into the water so that a light foaming action comes when spraying the floors and walls. Leave this until the foaming subsides, and rinse again. If the foaming action recurs, then the areas which still foam are not clean. Either raise the peroxide level of the original rinse water or merely respray the areas still contaminated with the mix until no more foaming occurs.

For an udder wash use 1 oz of 35% hydrogen peroxide to a gallon of warm water. The cows tend to have softer teats and are freer of bacteria on the teat ends which helps to keep down bacteria in the bulk tank.

To hold colostrum milk from spoilage until it is all fed to the newborn calf (depending on the time of year, pH of the milk, temperature, etc.) you can use from one-fourth ounce 35% hydrogen peroxide up to one ounce per gallon of colostrum milk.

For newborn calves To add extra oxygen, add 10 to 15 drops 35% hydrogen peroxide to a bottle of milk, morning and evening, per calf. This has helped to brighten up calves and cleans up some cases of scours.

A drench can be given for high fever and off-their-feed cows with mastitis, depending on the situation and case. Mix 1 to 2 ounces of 35% hydrogen peroxide to one quart of water, drenching the animal morning and evening for as long as needed, usually 2-3 days.

Ailing cows Use one pint of 3% hydrogen peroxide to five gallons of water.

Clean animal wounds with 3% hydrogen peroxide.

Induce vomiting in animals with 3% hydrogen peroxide as needed.

After birth of calves farmers have reported that their cows settle and clean out faster after giving birth to a calf when hydrogen peroxide is added to their drinking water.

Converting crop residue to cattle feed Hydrogen peroxide has also been used in converting crop residue into cattle feed. This could be an asset for the farmer, especially in times of drought. It is possible to take straw, cornstocks, corn cobs, soy bean residue, sawdust or even ground-up brush and use it for feed after treatment. By treating these materials with a weak solution of hydrogen peroxide, they can be turned into animal feed. The experimental work has been done by Michael Gould, US Department of Agriculture at Peoria, Illinois. The feedlot says the meat is reportedly as good as corn fed.

As I understand the process, they take a 1% solution of hydrogen peroxide and soak the residue for sixteen hours. This breaks down the fiber so that it can be assimilated. According to one article in the April 1986 issue of <u>FARM INDUSTRY NEWS</u>, Vol 19, No 4, they have taken wheat straw and, after treatment, ground it into flour and made tasty bread, cakes and pancakes with it. **To make a 1% solution, mix 1 part 35% food grade hydrogen peroxide to 34 parts water.**

Hogs In the production of hogs, it has been found that the meat is more lean when hydrogen peroxide is added to their drinking water. One hog raiser, who sells by grade and yield only, reported that he got the highest grade ever. Another raised one hog to 250 pounds for her own use. It yielded only 23 pounds of lard.

Another hog farmer took two hogs to be slaughtered for his own personal use. While there, the Federal Meat Inspector came and inspected his hogs. He was amazed to see how large the lungs were in comparison to another hog which was grown in close confinement. The latter hog had pneumonia, like most hogs raised this way. The pneumonia is held in check with antibiotics. The meat inspector told the farmer that his hogs were getting the proper amount of oxygen. "It takes oxygen to make good lean meat", he said. He then asked the farmer, "What are you doing?" The reply was, "I just treat the water with hydrogen peroxide."

Hogs with scours In the case of hogs with scours, use 100 ppm in water supply for 2-3 days, then back down to the normal amount, 20-30 ppm (use test trips to determine the actual amount in drinking water).

Slurry tanks A slurry tank is an outdoor tank where farmers store the animal waste from their dairy barns and/or hog operations. In Pennsylvania it has been found that by adding 15 gallons of 35% hydrogen peroxide to 350,000 gallons of slurry and agitating it, there is no odor given off from the slurry. Then a truckload tank of blackstrap molasses and bacteria is added several days prior to applying the slurry to their fields. Once again they put in 15 gallons of 35% hydrogen peroxide and agitate it. This is then applied on their fields for fertilizer. They have found that there is no odor and it is the finest liquid fertilizer they have ever used.

Chickens In the fall of 1983, over 1,000,000 chickens were given hydrogen peroxide in their drinking water because of the avian flu epidemic. None of these birds got the flu but before the epidemic was over, 11,000,000 chickens had to be destroyed and were put in a landfill.

A chicken farmer in eastern Ohio, with a flock of 20,000 egg layers, found that by putting hydrogen peroxide in their drinking water, the egg production went up 1,000 eggs per day. We now have a farmer raising 350,000 laying chickens on hydrogen peroxide with similar results.

A chicken raiser who raises heavy chickens said the problem she usually has had with the chicken's legs and tendons breaking was greatly decreased after using hydrogen peroxide in their drinking water. She also noticed when she dressed the chickens there were no breast blisters.

I am currently eating broilers raised on hydrogen peroxide and think they are the best chickens I have eaten since I was a small child. If we buy chickens from the supermarket, I rinse or soak them in a 3% dilute solution first to rid them of possible salmonella.

Decontamination of broiler carcasses Hydrogen peroxide was used experimentally at the rate of .5% to 1%, soaking the carcasses in this solution for ten minutes as a decontaminate for salmonella. The work was done in the Netherlands and published in 1987 POULTRY SCIENCE, Issue 66, pp 1555-1557.

Turkeys A number of turkey raisers throughout the US and Canada are using hydrogen peroxide in their drinking water. A turkey raiser in Canada put 20,000 turkeys on hydrogen peroxide. In the same growing time, they averaged one & one-half pounds more per bird, used 8 1/2% less feed and the mortality rate went down.

In Missouri a turkey raiser told me he took his turkeys from chicks to market without any medication or antibiotics. One of the head veterinarians of the State of Missouri was asked about the use of hydrogen peroxide in the drinking water of turkeys. His comment was, "It's only water and oxygen and cannot hurt them. It will not show up in the chemical residue test." This same farmer was awarded the *Grower of the Month* award.

A turkey grower in Wisconsin told me after using hydrogen peroxide on his turkeys that his chemical residue test came back with zero chemical residue.

Birds Hydrogen peroxide and sodium perborate were used by Robert Stroud to heal birds. He wrote about it in the book, *DISEASES OF BIRDS* which should be available at your local library. Stroud was the famous "Bird Man of Alcatraz."

Crops, Orchards & Plants

Foliar feed To foliar feed crops, put sixteen ounces of 35% food grade hydrogen peroxide into 20 gallons of water. This is sufficient for one acre. Spray on plants early in the morning for best results. (Did you know that the singing of the birds in the morning stimulates the opening of the pores of plants?)

Seed Germination To germinate seeds, put 1-3 ounces of 3% hydrogen peroxide into a pint of distilled water. Soak the seeds for 8 hours. An experiment was done soaking old wheat seeds with the solution, while also testing controlled seeds in plain water. The hydrogen peroxide-treated seeds germinated at a rate of 90%, while the controlled seeds germinated at a rate of 60%.

Insecticide Use hydrogen peroxide as an insecticide by mixing eight or more ounces of 3% hydrogen peroxide to a gallon of water with eight ounces of blackstrap molasses or white sugar. It has been found that the blackstrap molasses works better than sugar. It seems to adhere to the plant better. Spray as needed.

House & garden plants Use one ounce of the 3% hydrogen peroxide to a quart of water. Mist the plants with this solution and also spray on the ground in which they are planted.

Orchards Orchard owners are watering the ground around the trees using six to eight ounces of 3% hydrogen peroxide to a gallon of water. This solution can also be used as a spray. It has been reported that a pear tree that never bore fruit is now bearing after treatment.

Rice paddies Non-productive rice paddies have been reactivated by using the above formula.

Fish Farms Hydrogen peroxide is being used to disinfect water at fish farms so as to reduce the fungal growth on fish. Hydrogen peroxide is being put in the make-up water at the rate of 5 ppm. Tropical fish raisers have found that adding one ounce of 35% food grade hydrogen peroxide to 20 galup residence, they use what DNA (cellular blueprint) and RNA material there is available to reproduce themselves. This occurs on a massive, explosive scale and once they have exhausted their host's resources, they leave, looking for new debilitated, weak cells to invade. If they find, and are able to invade a sufficient quantity of these weakened cells, they become so great in number that their metabolic waste products begin to overwhelm our ability to detoxify them and various diseases result.

Ozone will act as a beneficial scavenger (all of Nature has such cleanup crews) by producing hydroxyperoxides which will efficiently destroy the diseased cell as well as the invading organisms through the oxidation reduction system we discussed before. Let me clarify hydroxyperoxides, because someone is sure to attack them as dangerous "free radicals" and mislead you.

I do not have the space to elaborate, but I am not totally convinced at this time (although I once was) that the present widely touted 'bad free radical' concept is totally accurate. Let me just say that the possibility exists that free radicals do not harm normal cells, but merely attack and destroy sick cells which are a detriment to the general health of the body. I believe that hydroxyperoxides actually enhance the health of strong cells by providing an additional source of oxygen to their environment.

The schematic on the next page reflects my concept of how this beneficial housecleaning action of the hydroxyperoxides formed by ozone takes place.

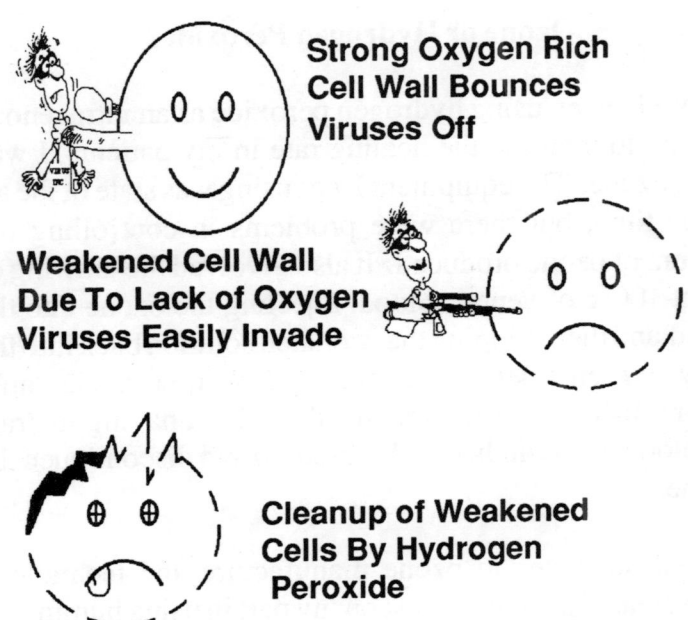

All of us should seek after the truth. The above schematic is by no means a proven fact. It does represent a plausible theory based upon what is known about hydroxyperoxide free radicals and their actions toward unfit cells and unwanted organisms. We must always remain mentally flexible enough to receive new information as it surfaces. The excellent clinical response to ozone therapy is a powerful ally in the above theory.

Ozone or Hydrogen Peroxide?

Before I began using hydrogen peroxide as an intravenous therapy to increase the healing rate in my patients, I was using ozone. The equipment I was using was state of the art at the time, but there were problems in controlling the amount of ozone produced. It also involved the drawing of about 100cc of venous blood, injecting the ozone into the blood and then dripping the ozonated solution back into the body. When I determined that hydrogen peroxide could accomplish much the same result without having to draw the blood, we switched to this method and discontinued the ozone.

Recent advances in ozone manufacture and technology have created a great interest on my part in using humidified ozone by rectal insufflation. The methodology allows repeated treatment during the day without invasive procedures such as required to give an intravenous infusion. The rectal tip is introduced and a thirty-second burst of humidified ozone is injected into the rectum, yielding about one-half liter. It is very painless and the reports I have seen indicate that a higher concentration of oxygen can be achieved in the blood stream by this method than by injecting the ozone directly into the boodstream. Our patients love it because there is almost always a feeling of well-being immediately after the treatment. We use this up to three times per day in critical patients. This treatment method is unique in that it avoids the intestinal cramps that injecting dry ozone into the rectum causes.

Summary

1) **Oxygen Depletion** In the not too distant past, the oxygen concentration in the air was approximately 38%. Due to any number of circumstances, which may include atomic experimentation and warfare, our worldwide industrialization and the oxygen-producing greenery such as forests, we are now at a level just over 19% - or half that which man used to enjoy. Evolution has not had time to expand our lung capacity or our ability to extract oxygen more efficiently, so we are conceivably in a constant state of oxygen deficiency.

2) **Resistance to Disease** It is rather well-known that viruses are "anaerobic" creatures which thrive in the absence of oxygen. The oxidation reduction system in the body which is our prime means of detoxification relies on a plentiful supply of oxygen to perform its function. When there is a deficiency of oxygen, unwanted organisms flourish and we wallow in our own waste products. In recent times our society has suffered from more persistent and tenacious organisms than ever before. We also have the highest rate of degenerative diseases ever.

3) **Hydrogen Peroxide, Magnesium Dioxide & Ozone Offer a Therapeutic Solution** The use of these three approaches to increasing the internal oxygen environment may be a solution that should be investigated. The response to all of these methods is often miraculous. Contrary to

the alleged bad effects that are produced by their use, clinical use has proven their value and safety. The oral use of magnesium dioxide and/or the drinking of ozonated water may be one of the real saving procedures for those who wish to enjoy better health. The intravenous use of hydrogen peroxide and the rectal insufflation of humidified ozone may be the greatest medical discoveries of the 1980's.

I am obviously very enthusiastic about this approach to disease. It avoids the chemical poisons which are characteristic of the allopathic philosophy and which often precipitate further illness. Nature's tools are usually the best.

For further information on oxygen therapies, please consider the book **OXYGEN THERAPIES** by Ed McCabe. This book is available from:

BOOKS
4100 Bonita Rd.
Bonita, Calif. 91902

Send $12 plus $2 shipping and handling.

Bibliography

1. Shenep JL, Stokes DC, Hughes WT: Lack of Antibacterial Activity After Intravenous Hydrogen Peroxide Infusion in Experimental Escherichia coli Sepses. Infect Immun 1985; 48; 607-610

2. Dockrell HM and Playfair JH: Killing of Blood-Stage Murine Malaria Parasites by Hydrogen Peroxide. Infect Immun 1983; 39: 456-459

3. Weiss SJ, Young J, Lo Buglio A, et al: Role of Hydrogen Peroxide in Neutriphil-Meiated Destruction of Cultured Endothelial Cells. J Clin Invest 1981; 68: 714-721

4. Root RK, Metcalf JA, Oshion N, et al: H2O2 Release from Human Granulocytes during Phagocytosis. J Clin Invest 1975; 55: 945-955

5. Root RK, Metcalf JA, Oshion N, et al: H2O2 Release from Human Granulocytes during Phagocytosis. J Clin Invest 1977; 60: 1266-1279

6. Takasashi M Hasegawa R, Furukawa F, et al: Effects of Ethanol, Potassium Metabisulfite, Formaldehyde and Hydrogen Peroxide on Gastric Carcinogenesis in Rats after Initiation with N-Methyl-N-Nitro-N-Nitrosoguandine. Jpn J Cancer Res 1986; 77 (2): 188-124

7. Jay BE, Finney JW, Balla GA, et al: The Supersaturation of Biologic Fluids with Oxygen by the Decomposition of Hydrogen Peroxide. Texas Rpts Biol & Med 1964; 22: 106-109

8. Balla GA, Finney JW, Aronoff BL, et al: Use of Intra-arterial Hydrogen Peroxide to Promote Would Healing. Am J Surg 1964; 108: 621-629

9. Fuson FL, Hylstra JA, Hochstein P, et al: Intravenous Hydrogen Peroxide Infusion as a Means of Extrapulmonary Oxygenation. Clin Res 1967; 15:74

10. MacNaughton JI: Regional Oxygenation & Radiotherapy: A Study of the Degradation of Infused Hydrogen Peroxide. II. Measurement of Decomposition of H2O2 Infused Into Flowing Blood. Int J Radiat Biol 1971; 19:415-426

11. Finney & Experimental Animals Following the Infusion of Hydrogen Peroxide into the Carotid Artery. Angio 1965; 16: 62-66

12. Mallams JT, Finney JW, and Balla GA: The Use of Hydrogen Peroxide As A Source of Oxygen in A Regional Intra-Arterial Infusion System. So MJ 1962; 55: 230-232

13. Urschel HC Jr: Cardiovascular Effects of Hydrogen Peroxide: Current Status. Dis of Chest 1967; 51: 180-192

14. Lorincz Al, Jacoby JJ, Livingstone MM: Studies on the Parenteral Administration of Hydrogen Peroxide. Anesthesiology 1948; 9: 162-174

15. Johnson RJR, Froese G, Khodadad M et al: Hydrogen Peroxide & Radiotherapy. Bubble Formation in Blood. Br J Radiol 1968; 41: 749-754

16. MacNaughton JI: Regional Oxygenation & Radiotherapy: A Study of the Degradation of Infused Hydrogen Peroxide. I. Infusate Mixing. Int J Radiat Biol 1971; 19: 405-413

17. Finney JW, Jay Be, Race GJ, et al: Removal of Cholesterol and Other Lipids from Experimental Animal and Human Atheromatous Arteries by Dilute Hydrogen Peroxide. Angiology 1966; 17: 223-228

18. Snyder LM, Fortier NL, Trainor J, et al: Effect of Hydrogen Peroxide Exposure on Normal Human Erythrocyte Deformability, Cross-linking. J Clin Invest 1985; 76: 1971-1977

19. Finney JW, Balla GA, Race GJ, et al: Peripheral Blood Changes in Humans & Experimental Animals Following the Infusion of Hydrogen Peroxide into the Carotid Artery. Angio 1965; 16: 62-66

20. Ackerman NB, Brinkley FB: Comparison of Effects on Tissue Oxygenation of Hyperbaric Oxygen & Intravascular Hydrogen Peroxide. Sur 1968; 63: 285-290

21. Germon PA, Faust DS, Brady, LW: Comparison of Arterial and Tissue Oxygen Measurements in Humans Receiving Regional Hydrogen Peroxide Infusions & Oxygen Inhalation. Radiology 1968; 91: 669-672

22. Lebedev LV, Levin AO, Romankova MP, et al: Regional Oxygenation in the Treatment of Severe Destructive Forms of Obliterating Diseases of the Extremity Arteries. Vestn Khir 1984; 132: 85-88

23. Urschel HC, Finney JW, Dull LM, et al: Treatment of Artheriosclerotic Obstructive Cerebrovascular Disease with Hydrogen Peroxide. Vas Surg 1967; 1: 77-81

24. Finney JW, Urschel HC, Balla GA, et al: Protection of the Ischemic Heart with DMSO Alone or DMSO with Hydrogen Peroxide. Ann NY Acad Sci 1967; 151: 231-241

25. Urschel HC, Finney JW, Morale AR, et al: Cardiac Resuscitation with Hydrogen Peroxide. Circ 1965; 31 (suppl II): II-210

26. Nathan CV and Cohn ZA: Antitumor Effects of Hydrogen Peroxide in Vivo. J Exp Med 1981; 154: 1553

27. Butler BD, and Hill BA: The Lungs as a Filter for Microbubbles. J Appl Physiol Respirat Environ Exercise Physiol 1979; 47(3): 537-543

28. Bate H: The Decomposition of Hydrogen Peroxide Infused into Flowing Blood. Int J Radiat Biol 1972; 22: 395-396

29. Crane D, Haussinger D, Sies H: Rise of Coenzyme A-Glutathione Mixed Disulfide during Hydroperpoxide Metabolism in Perfused Rat Liver. Euo J Biochem 1982; 127: 575-578

30. Wrigglesworth JM: Formation and Reduction of a 'Peroxy' Intermediate of Cytochrome cop Hydrogen Peroxide. Biochem J 1984; 217: 705-719

31. Levine PH, Weinger RS, Simon J, et al: Release of Hydrogen Peroxide by Granulocytes as a Modulator of cop platelet Reastions. J Clin Invest 1976; 57: 955-963

32. Polgar P, Taylor L. Stimuation of Prostaglandin Synthesis by Ascorbic Acid via Hydrogen Peroxide Formation. Prostag 1980; 19: 693

Dr. Christiaan Barnard Joins In Search For The Fountain Of Youth!

From the Seattle Times / Seattle Post-Intelligencer: Sunday, April 6, 1986:

" NEW YORK - Who knows? It could be the result of those fetal-lamb-cell injections administered at a chi-chi clinic in Switzerland. <u>Or maybe it's the hydrogen-peroxide tonic he swigs three times each day.</u> If that sounds too off the wall, you might chalk it up simply to retirement and the fact that after years of doing such dicey pioneer surgery as human heart transplants, the grind of the operating room is behind him. Then again, the man could just have a lot of zesty genes. Whatever the reason, Christiaan Barnard looks marvelous.

Tanned and trim, with nary a telltale wisp of gray at the temples or a trace of a crow's foot, South Africa's one-time medical meteor hardly blinks when people insist that he cannot be 63. "I do everything possible," he replies matter-of factly, "to retard the aging process."

OKLAHOMA HEART CENTER
3300 Northwest Expressway
Oklahoma City, Oklahom 73112
(405)-949-3349

March 10, 1986

Mr. John F. Wright
Northam House
Saltern Way Lilliput
Poole Dorset BH14 8 JR
England

Dear Mr. Wright:

Thank you for your letter of February 25, 1986. It is true I have found relief from the arthritis and I attribute this to taking hydrogen peroxide orally several times each day. I learned of this treatment from Mr. Walter Grotz and suggest that you could possibly write to him for further data regarding this treatment.

Best wishes,

Christiaan N. Barnard, M.D., Ph.D.*

cc: Walter Grotz

* **Signature On File**

GRADES OF HYDROGEN PEROXIDE

3% Hydrogen Peroxide (Drug/Grocery variety)
Made from 50% Super D Peroxide, Diluted. Contains stabilizers - phenol, acetanilide, sodium stanate and Tetrasodium phosphate among them.

6% Hydrogen Peroxide (used by Beauticians)
Comes in strengths labeled 10, 20 and 40 volume. Must have an activator added to be used as a bleach. Do not consume.

30% Re-Agent Hydrogen Peroxide
Used in Medical research. Also contains stabilizers.

30-32% Electronic Grade Hydrogen Peroxide
Used for washing transistors and integrated chip parts before assembly. Stabilizers contained are unknown.

35% Technical Grade Hydrogen Peroxide
Contains a small amount of phosphorus to neutralize any chlorine in the water it is combined with.

35% Food Grade Hydrogen Peroxide
Used in food products like cheese, eggs, whey products. Also used to spray inside of foil lined containers for food storage - known as the aseptic packaging system. The product of choice in most applications using hydrogen peroxide.

90% Hydrogen Peroxide
Used by the Military as a source of Oxygen at Cape Canaveral. Used as a propulsion source in rocket fuel.

Simple Treatment for Warts
Cumulated Index Medicus, 1962
(An Easy and Painless Treatment of Warts)

It is difficult to find a wart treatment which pleases everyone, doesn't leave scars, and allows one to continue working normally while undergoing treatment. Cutting, burning and freezing them are the accepted treatment, but often are unsuitable since they are too bloody, painful or leave scars behind.

We have perfected a means of removing warts using a well researched disinfectant - Hydrogen Peroxide. The technique is very easy. One needs a sharp spoon, not to remove the wart, but to open the surface of the wart by gently scraping. Do not cause bleeding by excessive scraping. Apply one drop of 35% hydrogen peroxide onto the opened surface and let dry. After 2 days, scrape off the dried layer and add another drop of hydrogen peroxide. After the application the patient will feel at most a prickly sensation which will last a few minutes. After that it could itch, but this also disappears after a short time.

The many patients we have treated with this have had uniform good results. It will usually take from 2 to 10 applications, depending on the size of the wart. When it vanishes, it is gone without a trace - no scar!

July 8, 1988

Greetings To All Interested in Hydrogen Peroxide:

As you are well aware, I have been an outspoken advocate of hydrogen peroxide for several years. As such I have had to defend the properties of this rather simple but remarkable substance many times. One of the most difficult to defend was the obnoxious taste and aftertaste that occurs when used orally. Because I felt so deeply about the product and was so encouraged by its results, I embarked upon a search for a way in which the benefits of the free oxygen could be enjoyed without the nauseating flavor.

After two years and 30 some different attempts, I ran across the answer to the problem. I am well aware others have tried and, in fact, still are trying. Walter Grotz told me of a very wealthy man who had hired a chemist to try and do what we had done. **It is proprietary information! It is a trade secret! I am not going to divulge what I am doing!**

But I would like to say that I resent some of the accusations which have been presented by those who have been unable to compete. Let me present a few questions that should stop the innuendo:

1. I am very proud of my reputation and would not jeopardize such by chicanery in actually putting less oxygen in the product than I represent. Hydrogen peroxide is cheap. Yes, I do alter it in the process for this purpose and that

alteration has resulted in a very tasty, acceptable product. But do you think I would reduce an ingredient that costs pennies, plus misbrand a product???

2. There has never been a product that continued to sell that didn't please the customers; in other words, get results. Does it get results?? Hasn't it been one of the most enthusiastically received products in years??

3. I completely admit to being paranoid about my little secret and I'm not going to tell anyone about it. There would be 100 imitiators in three weeks. Am I wrong in protecting my own work??

Think about it!!

Kurt W. Donsbach, D.C., Ph.D.

> This letter was written three years ago during a period of time when many jealous people were making untrue statements about the special hydrogen peroxide formula I had developed. We now have the new improved magnesium peroxide formulas.

EMBRACING WHOLISTIC HEALTH

by Kurt W. Donsbach, D.C., N.D., Ph.D.

CLARIFYING THE BODY-MIND-SPIRIT CONNECTION in
CANCER • ARTHRITIS • CANDIDIASIS
HEART DISEASE • MULTIPLE SCLEROSIS

Explicit treatment protocols from the world famous natural healing institutions - Hospital Santa Monica, Hospital St. Augustine and Institut Santa Monica

You can order this 300 page profusely illustrated manual by checking with your local health food store or calling 1-800-423-7662. Total Cost: $14.95. Dr. Donsbach feels this is his best work yet. You should have this book on your shelf to help you answer health questions that may come up. It is the best review of the application and merits of wholistic health philosophy available today.

AL-DON UNIVERSITY

of

Wholistic Health Sciences Announces A Rare Educational Opportunity

- Progressive Off-Campus Study Programs
- Programs for Every Purpose:
  - Professional Service
  - Personal Enlightenment
  - Post Graduate Education
  - Hospital Internship Available

Founding Faculty:
Kurt W. Donsbach, D.C., N.D., Ph.D.
H. Rudolph Alsleben, M.D., D.O., Ph.D.
John Huffman, D.Sc., Ph.D.
Montross Pelton, Ph.D.
Mary Carter, R.N., Ph.D.
Albert LaRusch, D.C., N.D.
Arne Liss, Ph.D.

Certificates & Degrees Available

Call 1-619-475-2874 For Further Information

REACH FOR LIFE
HEALTH
SPA

A Luxurious Facility at Economy Prices
12 day programs starting at $1725

Supervised by
Kurt W. Donsbach, D.C., N.D., Ph.D.
H. Rudolph Alsleben, M.D., D.O., Ph.D.

Complete Physical Examination
Blood and Urine Analysis
Bio-Ionization Analysis
Nutrition Counseling
Chelation
Herbal Body Wraps
Pain Relief Therapy
Facial Rejuvenation
Live Cell Therapy
Juice Fasting
Massage and Physiotherapy

For Further Information Call: 1-800-359-6547